Seated Yoga for Seniors

Step-by-step Blueprint On How To Use Seated Yoga To Deal With Everyday Issues As A Senior

(©) 2024. Tina Casteel. All rights reserved.

This book or any portion thereof may not be reproduced or used in any manner whatsoever without the express written permission of the publisher except for the use of brief quotations in a book review.

Introduction

Have you come across some information that seated yoga will help you stretch your muscles without stressing your body, but you are hesitant because you do not know the exact steps to follow or how long you should exercise?

And would you like to have a comprehensive guide that will show you what seated/chair yoga and warm-up poses you can do, all with comprehensive steps and illustrations to crown it all?

If you have answered YES, keep reading...

Aging brings about health complications and ailments such as lung disorders, heart conditions, sore knees, back pain, and others that may make it challenging to engage in challenging and common exercises like push-ups, jumping jacks, and others. But even with these ailments and others that limit your normal movement, there is a type of exercise that can accommodate you: **seated/chair yoga!**

Seated yoga is one of the best exercise paradigms for seniors, thanks to its many benefits and beginner-friendliness.

If you've never done seated yoga, you might have questions like:

- *Why seated yoga?*
- *How long should I do the poses to avoid feeling pain?*
- *What different yoga poses can I do?*
- *If I feel pain while doing the poses, what can I do?*

If you have these and other similar questions, you are reading the right book that will answer these and other similar questions in easy-to-understand, simple language!

Here is a sneak peek of some of the key things you will learn from this book:

- **The basics of seated yoga:** What seated yoga is, its history, and proof that it indeed works

- **Seated warm-up exercises:** Different warm-up exercises to prepare your body for the main seated yoga exercises

- Different seated yoga exercises for seniors

- How to address any discomforts experienced while exercising

- **And much more!**

Before we dive right into the thick of it, please take a moment to imagine how great it would feel to stand up without feeling like your back is breaking!

With this image in mind, dive headlong into the first page to learn how your vision of a pain-free body can come true, all thanks to seated yoga.

Let us begin.

PS: I'd like your feedback. If you are happy with this book, please leave a review on Amazon.

Please leave a review for this book on Amazon by visiting the page below:

https://amzn.to/2VMR5qr

Table of Contents

Introduction 2

Chapter 1: Seated Yoga – The Basics 14

Chapter 2: Seated Yoga Warm-Up Exercises 17

Warm-up Variation 1 18

Warm-up Variation 2 18

Warm-up Variation 3 19

Warm-up Variation 4 20

Warm-up Variation 5 21

Chapter 3: Seated Yoga Exercises 23

Upper Body Seated Yoga Exercises 23

Seated Yoga Exercise 1: Overhead Stretch 24

Seated Yoga Exercise 2: Seated Mountain/Tadasana 31

Seated Yoga Exercise 3: Chair Spinal Twist 35

Seated Yoga Exercise 4: Cat-Cow Stretch 40

Seated Yoga Exercise 5: Reverse Arm Hold 45

Seated Yoga Exercise 6: Single-Leg Stretch/Head-To-Knee Pose (Janu Sirsasana) 51

Seated Yoga Exercise 7: Shoulder Press 57

Seated Yoga Exercise 8: Seated Front Shoulder Raises 61

Seated Yoga Exercise 9: Seated Chest Press 66

Seated Yoga Exercise 10: Isolated Tricep Extensions 71

Seated Yoga Exercise 11: Bicep Curls 75

Seated Yoga Exercise 12: Knee-to-Chest Pose 78

Seated Yoga Exercise 13: Seated Ts .. 81

Seated Yoga Exercise 14: Seated Leg Scissors 83

Seated Yoga Exercise 15: Seated Crunches 85

Seated Yoga Exercise 16: Seated Chest Opener 87

Lower Body Seated Yoga Exercises 90

Seated Yoga Exercise 17: Chair Warrior 91

Seated Yoga Exercise 18: Eagles Arms 95

Seated Yoga Exercise 19: Seated Forward Bend/ Paschimottanasana in Sanskrit 98

Seated Yoga Exercise 20: Marches. 103

Seated Yoga Exercise 21: Ankle Stretch 109

Seated Yoga Exercise 22: Extender Leg Raises Pose 112

Seated Yoga Exercise 23: Leg Kicks 115

Seated Yoga Exercise 24: Knee Extensions 119

Seated Yoga Exercise 25: Seated Hip Stretch................................123

Seated Yoga Exercise 26: Seated Pillow Squeeze Pose....................................126

Seated Yoga Exercise 27: Seated Clamshells..129

Seated Yoga Exercise 28: Seated Single-Leg Calf Raises.....................135

Seated Yoga Exercise 29: Seated Beanbags Yoga Pose Routine..........138

Seated Yoga Exercise 30: Seated Cow Face Pose 142

Chapter 4: Seated Yoga Poses: A Few Things to Note....................145

How often should you do seated yoga poses?..145

How long should a seated yoga session be? 146

Conclusion 147

Chapter 1: Seated Yoga – The Basics

Seated yoga is a type of yoga done while seated on a chair, bean bed, or couch. Like most seniors, you can attest that aging brings about many issues that leave us wishing we never moved from our chairs, right?

Well, as you will see from this book, this specific form of yoga is suitable for healthy seniors and any senior suffering from physical disabilities and, in our case, seniors who find standard yoga too challenging. Lakshmi Voelker, a renowned yoga teacher, created chair yoga around 1982.

Lakshmi Voelker did not come up with this form of yoga coincidentally. As she puts it, her doctors diagnosed her with arthritis that was so severe that she could no longer exercise as anyone would normally because she could not get down on the floor. Her predicament motivated her to develop a tangible sequence anyone can do comfortably on a chair.

Since 2005, Lakshmi has helped certify 1,500 yoga teachers nationally and internationally, which means this form of yoga really works!

Let's further prove how effective chair yoga is by discussing different studies:

A study done in 2016[1] investigated the effects of chair yoga on seniors; the study involved 42 respondents and a control group of 42 respondents. The results proved that chair yoga is a useful measure for prevention against functional decline in older adults. In addition, this study recommended chair yoga as a complementary practice for all nursing seniors!

---

[1] https://bit.ly/3CiQDog

Researchers at the Florida Atlantic University[2] did a study and published its results in an issue of the Journal of the American Geriatrics Society. The study sought to determine the effects of chair yoga on physical function and pain in older adults suffering from osteoarthritis.

The results revealed that seniors who engage in chair yoga experience a pain reduction lasting about three months after the poses! This means that the longer you do the poses (regularity matters), the less pain you will feel!

From the two studies and Lakshmi's story, you can see that there're no doubts about the effectiveness of chair/seated yoga. Next, let us get started by doing some warm-up exercises.

---

[2] https://www.sciencedaily.com/releases/2017/01/170111091417.htm

Chapter 2: Seated Yoga Warm-Up Exercises

As with any other type of exercise, engaging in warm-up exercises before doing the main exercises is essential for several reasons:

- Warm-up exercises increase the body temperature. Once the temperature rises, the muscle temperature rises, and oxygen flows more freely in the said muscles, making it possible to perform more complicated yoga poses without straining.

- Warm-up exercises also boost muscle elasticity. The elasticity factor is more important because more elastic muscles mean fewer occurrences of accidents or overheating.

So, with these benefits in mind, let us look at one of the main and most effective warm-up exercises.

Warm-up Variation 1

- Take a seat and sit up tall in your chair. Ensure your shoulders stay back and pulled downwards.

- Bring the head back.

- Look up to the ceiling and go back as far as you can. Be careful not to pull back in a way that causes you pain.

- Hold for a minimum of 60 seconds.

- And you are done!

Warm-up Variation 2

- Get a seat and sit up tall in a chair. Ensure the shoulders are pushed back and pulled down.

- Bring the chin down to the chest. Do not overdo this position because you should not feel any pain.

- Place your hands on the back of the head. Apply gentle pressure while doing this.

- Hold for 60 seconds.

- And you are done!

Warm-up Variation 3

- Get a seat and sit up tall. Ensure that your shoulders stay back and that you have them pulled downwards.

- Place your palms on the knees.

- Look over to one side. Turn your head as far as possible while being as comfortable as possible.

- For each head turn, hold that position for 60 seconds or more.

Warm-up Variation 4

- Get a seat and sit up tall. Ensure that your shoulders stay back and that you have them pulled downwards.

- Bring one ear down to the shoulder. Kindly do not bring the shoulder up to the ear. Instead, keep the shoulder in a relaxed position.

- Place one hand over the head, then apply some pressure.

- For each step, hold for a minimum of 60 seconds.

- After doing one side, switch to the other side.

- And you are done!

Warm-up Variation 5

- Get a seat and sit up tall. Ensure that your shoulders stay back and that you have them pulled downwards.

- Place one hand behind the shoulder, as seen in the first image above; go as back as you can and be keen not to feel any pain.

- Turn your head to roughly 45 degrees to one side.

- Bring the head down. The pose should have you look as if you are looking down at your knee.

- Hold this position for 60 seconds.

- Place your hand on the back of your head, then apply slight pressure.

- Hold this position for 60 seconds, then repeat the process on the opposite side.

And you are done with your warm-up session!

With this warm-up session, you are ready to get into the main poses! Let us discuss them next.

Chapter 3: Seated Yoga Exercises

To make these poses easier to navigate and use for different body parts, let's segment them into the following groupings:

Upper Body Seated Yoga Exercises

The following list of seated/chair exercises targets your upper body. With age, your body will undergo many changes that may negatively affect it.

Therefore, it is essential to work the upper body if you want to live a life full of coordination. With boosted coordination, you will have no problems doing simple activities such as turning and picking up things.

Seated Yoga Exercise 1: Overhead Stretch

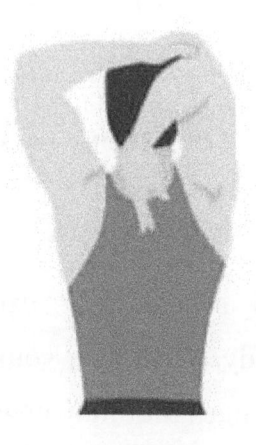

This pose will target the shoulders, lats, triceps, forearms, and chest, thereby working out most, if not all, of your entire upper body.

Specifically, this pose will help deal with the following:

- Chest pains from illnesses such as acute coronary syndrome, aortic dissection, and unstable pericarditis. Proof of this was in a study published in September 2020[3]. The study urged all who have chest issues to incorporate this exercise into their rehabilitation plan.

- Shoulder pains from rheumatoid disease, Milwaukee shoulder, and glenohumeral osteoarthritis. Proof of this was in a study done in 2016 titled "The effectiveness of a neck and shoulder stretching exercise program among office workers with neck pain: a randomized control trial."[4] This study proved that engaging in a stretching exercise like the overhead stretch for four weeks will decrease any shoulder and neck-related pain and improve their functions considerably!

---

[3] https://www.ncbi.nlm.nih.gov/pmc/articles/PMC7559714/
[4] https://bit.ly/3vI2Fn7

- Back and spine pain from illnesses like spinal cord injuries, tumors, herniated discs, bone disease, and arthritis. Harvard Health Publishing affirmed this in 2014 in an article titled "Stretching and strengthening are key to healing and preventing back pain."[5]

    This study-based article reports that stretching–in this case, through the overhead stretch–is a key way to deal with back pain recurrences.

- Arm pain from illnesses such as rotator cuff injury. Health and Safety Executive[6] published a research report to affirm this. In their report, the researchers made a case for using stretches (like the overhead stretch) to reduce arm pain as long as the exercise is repetitive and coupled with regular breaks.

---

[5] https://bit.ly/3vC3HkE
[6] https://www.hse.gov.uk/research/rrpdf/rr743.pdf

To do this pose, follow the steps below:

- First, warm-up.

- Next, get seated. Be as comfortable as possible.

- Next, place your arms down by your sides.

- Next, inhale one deep breath.

- Next, stretch your arms upwards to the sky. Hold this position for a minimum of 20 seconds or as long as you can hold your breath.

- Finally, exhale and bring down both hands.

As you do this exercise, there are a few things you should keep in mind, or rather, some basic mistakes you should do your best to avoid:

- Do not push your arms too far back: Doing this may lead to severe injuries such as muscle tears.

- Do not bounce your arms backward: This will cause tendon or muscle tears because you will have triggered a reaction within the muscle that will prevent the arms from relaxing as they should.

Once you get accustomed to this pose, move on to the next pose, which, to some extent, many liken to the overhead stretch pose.

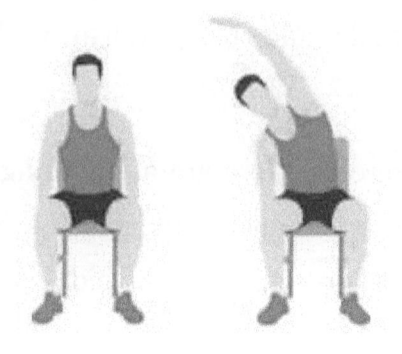

- First, warm-up.

- Get a seat and sit at the edge. Ensure that your back is upright and that the spine is straight. In addition, ensure that you have your feet firmly placed on the floor, with the lower body and the hips in a stable position.

- Using your right hand, grip the right side of your seat.

- Use the other hand–the left hand– to touch above the head. That will make a "C" shape or something similar to a spoon.

- Gently and slowly shift your upper torso to the right side. Keep the abdomen tight.

- Hold this position for 20 seconds, then shift to the other side.

- Finally, do 10 repetitions for each side to complete the exercise!

Mix the steps above with the steps below for more efficiency:

- First, warm-up.

- Get a seat and sit while keeping your feet flat on the floor, look forward, and keep your shoulders rolled back.

- Bend forward.

- Hinge from the waist. Ensure that you keep your back straight.

- Reach for the floor. To do this, bend while moving your legs apart. Hold this position for 10 seconds, then come back up.

- Do 5 sets of 20 repetitions, and you will be done!

Seated Yoga Exercise 2: Seated Mountain/Tadasana

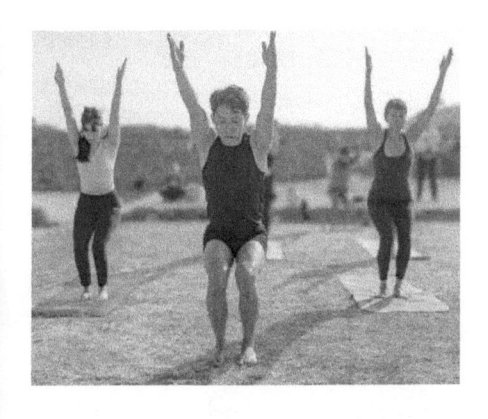

This pose will target your stomach and lower back muscles, enabling you to stand without slumping or slouching over. This pose will also elevate pains from illnesses associated with these two body parts:

- **Stomach/abdominal pain:** You will feel less pain and discomfort from illnesses such as peptic ulcer, appendicitis, constipation, IBS, and hernia. Proof of this is in a study titled "Irritable Bowel Syndrome: Yoga as

Remedial Therapy[7]." This study proved that yoga poses targeting the abdomen – like this one– will help relieve abdominal pain symptoms.

- **Lower back pain:** You will feel less pain and discomfort from illnesses such as facet joint and lumbar osteoarthritis, sacroiliac joint dysfunction, lumbar spinal stenosis, degenerative spondylolisthesis, and spinal compression fracture. Proof of this is in a study titled "Yoga as a treatment for chronic low back pain: A systematic review of the literature" done in 2016[8]. This study proves that yoga, in this case, the seated mountain yoga pose, will treat chronic low back pain. Specifically, it can

---

[7] https://www.ncbi.nlm.nih.gov/pmc/articles/PMC4438173/

[8] https://www.ncbi.nlm.nih.gov/pmc/articles/PMC4878447/

reduce chronic low back pain and can also reduce any disability that it may have caused.

To do this pose, follow the steps below;

- First, warm-up.

- Next, take a chair and sit on it. Be as comfortable as possible.

- Next, move/slide to the front half of your chair.

- Next, put your hands above the knees. Ensure that there is a small space between the knees. The space can be shoulder-width or slightly smaller.

- Next, place your palms on the knees as shown in the image above.

- Next, bend the knees to an angle of 90.

- Inhale slowly and hold the inhale for 5 seconds or more.

- Exhale while rolling your shoulders, then place your hands at the sides of the body, preferably at the waist.

- Finally, inhale and hold for 5 seconds or more, then exhale and hold for 5 seconds. Do 20 repetitions of this last step.

Seated Yoga Exercise 3: Chair Spinal Twist

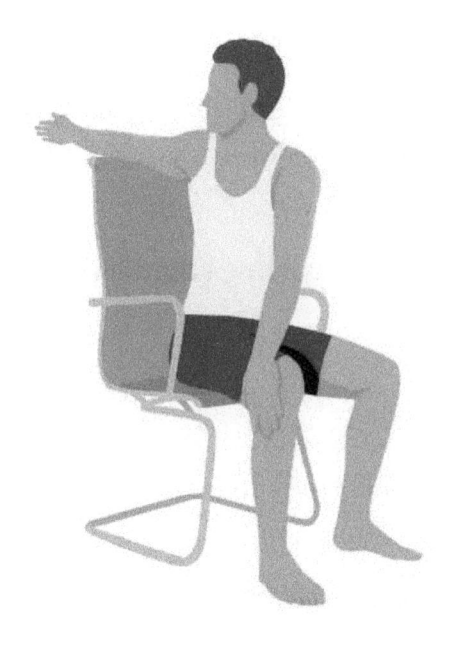

This pose targets the spine, belly, and back muscles. That makes it perfect for someone who wants to work on their upper body! This pose will also elevate pains from illnesses associated with these three body parts (we have mentioned what pains associate with the belly and spine in the previous poses, so let us discuss the last left):

- **Back muscles:** You will feel less pain and discomfort from lower back illnesses, which we have already discussed, and from upper back illnesses like kyphosis, frozen shoulder, adhesive capsulitis, tendinopathy, and the rotator cuff tear. Proof of this is in a study titled "Impact of yoga on low back pain and function: A systematic review and meta-analysis[9]." This study recommended that if you have back pain, doing 12 to 24 weeks of yoga poses and, in this case, the chair spinal twist, will reduce back pain and improve back pain function.

---

[9] https://www.researchgate.net/publication/256096645_Impact_of_Yoga_on_Low_Back_Pain_and_Function_A_Systematic_Review_and_Meta-Analysis#:~:text=Moreover%2C%20the%20improvements%20in%20pain,chronic%20low%20back%20pain%20patients.

To do this pose, follow the steps below;

- First, warm-up.

- Next, get a seat and sit on it.

- Next, move/slide to the side and sit, as seen in the image above.

- While at the side, slide to the back—you should be to the side of the right arm. At this juncture, ensure that your back is as straight as possible.

- Hold the back of the chair with both hands. This may be difficult, especially if you have issues with the upper back but try to reach it.

- While in the previous position, inhale deeply. Hold this position for a minimum of 5 seconds. Increase this time as you get accustomed to this pose.

- Next, gently and slowly turn your body towards the back of the chair. Do not overexert yourself here. With time, you will be able to go further and further back. When you reach your end, inhale for a minimum of 5 seconds, then exhale for another 5 seconds.

- Do 10 repetitions of the last step.

- After completing the steps above, rest for 2 minutes, switch to the other side and repeat the steps we have discussed.

There is also another way to do this same exercise. Find the steps for this alternative method below:

- First, warm-up.

- Get a couch and sit down.

- Get a pillow and twist side to side from the waist—ensure that you do not do this from the neck. When you reach your end, inhale again for a minimum of 5 seconds, then exhale for another 5 seconds.

- Do 10 repetitions of the last step.

- After completing these steps, rest for 2 minutes, switch to the other side and repeat the steps.

- And you are done!

Seated Yoga Exercise 4: Cat-Cow Stretch

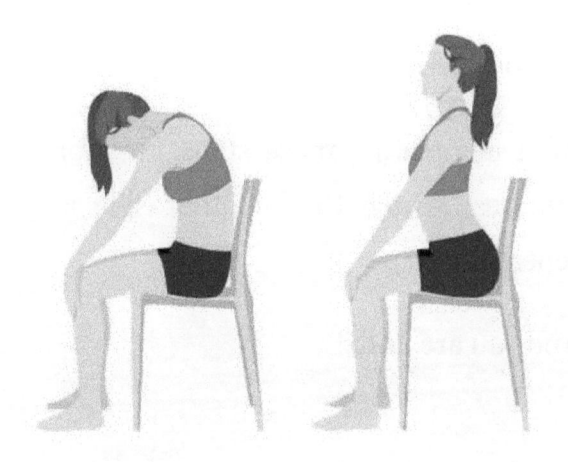

This pose will target your back, abdomen, hips, lungs, and chest. It will also alleviate pains and tension from illnesses associated with these five body parts:

- **Hips:** You will feel less pain and discomfort from hip illnesses and disorders such as bone fractures, ankylosing spondylitis, rheumatoid arthritis, and osteoarthritis. Researchers conducted a study to assess if yoga can help address hip illnesses and disorders. The results of this 2021 study[10] proved that it could reduce hip pain, improve hip function and quality of life, reduce depression, and help reduce serious adverse hip complications.

- **Chest and lungs:** You will feel less pain and discomfort from chest and lungs illnesses and disorders such as interstitial lung disease, pneumoconiosis, pleural effusion, pneumonia, acute respiratory distress syndrome, pulmonary hypertension, pulmonary edema, tuberculosis, cystic fibrosis, lung cancer, emphysema, acute bronchitis, chronic bronchitis, chronic

---

[10] https://www.ncbi.nlm.nih.gov/pmc/articles/PMC8459826/

compulsive pulmonary disease, and asthma.

To affirm this, researchers did a study titled "Exploring the therapeutic effects of yoga and ability to increase quality of life[11]." The results proved that yoga poses, in this case, the cat-cow stretch, will enhance your muscular strength, body flexibility, respiratory and cardiovascular function and reduce stress, depression, anxiety, and chronic pain. In addition, this pose will improve your sleep patterns and enhance your overall well-being! This study was under a body called Johns Hopkins Medicine[12]. This body noted that regular yoga practice can considerably lower stress levels and help with recovery from

---

[11] https://www.ncbi.nlm.nih.gov/pmc/articles/PMC3193654/
[12] https://www.hopkinsmedicine.org/health/wellness-and-prevention/the-yoga-heart-connection

different lung and heart illnesses and disorders.

To do this pose, follow the steps below;

- First, warm-up.

- Next, get a seat and sit on it.

- Next, slide to the edge of the chair. While in this position, ensure your back is as straight as possible.

- Next, inhale and arch your back as far back as possible. This will be the cow pose portion of this whole pose.

- Next, hold your breath 5 times for 5 seconds minimum each while in this position.

- Next, go back to the original position and invert the arch. To do this, have your shoulders align above the hips and the back curve forward.

- At this juncture, hold the position for 5 breaths that last for 5 seconds minimum each
- Finally, go to the original position.
- Do 10 repetitions

Seated Yoga Exercise 5: Reverse Arm Hold

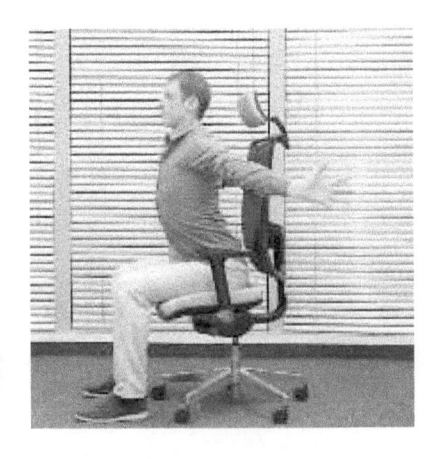

This pose targets your collarbone, shoulder, wrist, forearm, hands, and chest. Therefore, this pose will elevate pains and tension from illnesses associated with these six body parts:

- **Collarbone:** You will feel less pain and discomfort from collarbone illnesses and disorders such as broken collarbone, osteomyelitis, cancer (specifically Ewing's sarcoma), distal clavicular osteolysis, osteoarthritis, and thoracic outlet syndrome. Proof of this is in a study titled "Effects of yoga on patients with chronic nonspecific neck pain" done in 2019[13]. The study concluded that doing yoga that focuses on or targets the neck will always positively affect any neck-related pain.

- **Forearm:** You will feel less pain and discomfort from forearm illnesses and disorders such as polymyalgia rheumatica, sarcopenia, carpal tunnel syndrome, inclusion body myositis, and Paget's disease of bone. Proof of this is in a study titled "Can yoga have any effect on shoulder and arm pain and quality of life in patients with breast cancer? A randomized, controlled single-blind

---

[13] https://www.ncbi.nlm.nih.gov/pmc/articles/PMC6407933/#:~:text=The%20results%20show%20that%20yoga,Z%20%3D%203.95%2C%20P%20%3C%20.

trial[14]." This study proves that if you have arm pain due to other illnesses, doing yoga poses, and in this case, the reverse arm hold pose, will help reduce forearm-related pains after two and a half months of consistent exercising.

- **Hands:** You will feel less pain and discomfort from hand illnesses and disorders such as osteoarthritis, ganglion cysts, Dupuytren's disease, trigger finger, arthritis, and carpal tunnel syndrome. Proof of this comes to us thanks to the John Hopkins Arthritis Center through their 2018 publication[15]. This article says that yoga poses like the reverse arm hold is perfect for boosting joint health.

---

[14] https://www.sciencedirect.com/science/article/abs/pii/S1744388117304073

[15] https://www.hopkinsarthritis.org/patient-corner/disease-management/yoga-for-arthritis/

To do this pose, follow the steps below:

- First, warm-up.

- Sit down on a chair and slide straight to the edge.

- Have your arms at the side of your body, then inhale. Ensure you have your palms facing down. Hold your breath for 5 seconds minimum.

- While exhaling, roll your shoulders forward, and then roll your palms until you have them facing each other. Please note that at first, go as far as you can – the arms do not have to face each other immediately. Hold this position for a minimum of 5 seconds. After a while, you will be able to do it.

- And you are done!

If the steps above seem too complicated, you can follow the steps below;

- First, warm up.

- Spread your feet. You can do the shoulder-width distance.

- Take the left arm, then take it behind you and direct it towards the right arm.

- Interlace the two arms. Remember, the left arm will have traveled to the other hand while the right arm will just bend slightly to hold the left arm (you will have to bend the arm at an angle of 90 degrees or slightly less).

- Pull the left arm to the front.

- When you interlace your fingers, I suggest that if you begin on the left, remember to do the same to the right. This will balance the sternum pull.

- Finally, to make it easier to take your hands behind you easily without feeling pain, you should start by lifting your shoulders, bending your elbows, and then swinging your hands in the back.

Seated Yoga Exercise 6: Single-Leg Stretch/Head-To-Knee Pose (Janu Sirsasana)

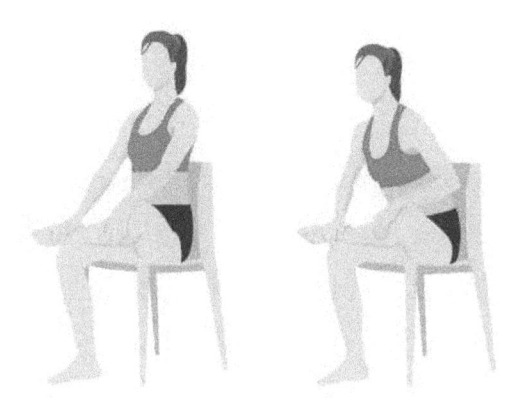

This pose will target your abdominal muscles, neck, groin, shoulders, and hamstrings.

Therefore, this pose will elevate pains and tension from illnesses associated with these five body parts:

- **Abdominal muscles:** You will feel less pain and discomfort from abdominal illnesses and disorders such as dementia, myasthenia gravis, multiple sclerosis, stroke, and diabetes. Proof of this is in a study done in 2014 titled "Core muscle during specific yoga poses[16]." This study affirms that yoga poses targeting the abdomen will strengthen the core if you do them correctly. This means your abdomen will be healthy and strong enough to weather any pain.

- **Groin:** You will feel less pain and discomfort from groin illnesses and disorders such as knee pains, Legg-calve-Perthes disease, urinary tract infection, inflammatory bowel disease, pelvic inflammatory disease,

---
[16] https://www.sciencedirect.com/science/article/abs/pii/S0965229914000107

endometriosis, inguinal hernia, and other abdominal hernias. Proof of this is in a study done in 2012 titled "Effect of yoga therapy in reversible inguinal hernia: A quasi-experimental study[17]." This study proves that adopting yoga directed to different body parts, such as this one that targets the groin, will help make the groin healthier. This study encourages you to adopt this yoga pose because it might help treat severe illnesses such as reversible inguinal hernia.

To do this pose, follow the steps below;

- First, do a warm-up set.

- Please take a seat and sit at its edge.

---

[17] https://www.ncbi.nlm.nih.gov/pmc/articles/PMC3276927/

- Have your feet at shoulder width distance.

- Lift one leg and fold it on the chair, as shown in the image above. The knee should stay suspended in the air.

- Bring the shoulders and head to rest on the folded knee, as shown in the image above, then tightly hug your knee, take a big breath in, and hold for a minimum of 5 seconds or more.

- If you have rested one leg on the other, ensure you release your hands and have them hanging freely by your side. Then, while inhaling, gently bend the back, shoulders, and head as much as possible and for as long as possible. You can begin with 5 seconds.

- Release, then switch the legs and repeat the process above.

Here is another variation you can try;

- First, do a warm-up set.

- Take a chair and sit at the edge.

- Stretch out one of your legs until that leg's heel rests on the floor while its toes face upwards.

- Take your arms and rest them on the outstretched leg.

- Inhale and exhale for a total of 10 breaths minimum or more.

- Inhale again, then bend over the outstretched leg (slide your arms downwards as you bend down).

- There is no specific distance regarding how far you should bend. Ideally, start slow and then intensify the bend as you get accustomed to this pose.

- While bent, inhale and exhale as slowly as possible for a total of 5 breaths or more.

- Finally, repeat these steps with the other leg.

- Interchange the legs around 10 times— for starters.

Seated Yoga Exercise 7: Shoulder Press

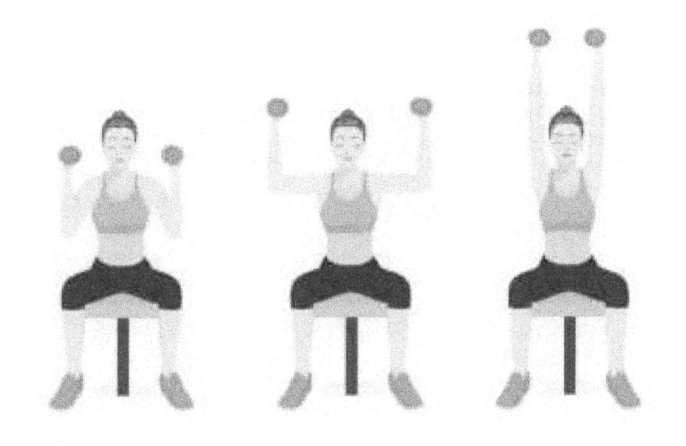

This pose will target your shoulders. Specifically, this pose will target your pectoralis major, medial deltoid, and anterior deltoid muscles. That means the pose will help address issues such as acute rotator cuff tear (also known as shoulder arthritis), rheumatoid arthritis, tendonitis, osteoarthritis, frozen shoulder, and bursitis, among others.

Several studies prove that this pose will help make your shoulder better. For example, we have a study conducted in 2016 titled "The effects of yoga on shoulder and spinal actions for women with breast cancer-related lymphoedema of the arm: A randomized controlled pilot study.[18]"

This study proves that eight weeks of yoga—in this case, shoulder press—will improve the lumbopelvic posture. In addition, it will boost your shoulder abduction, especially if you have any illness or disorder affecting your arm.

Another 2018 study titled "The use of medical therapeutic yoga on a patient with adhesive capsulitis: A case report[19]" also proves that yoga (in this case, the shoulder press) poses will help make your shoulder better. This study's results

---
[18] https://www.ncbi.nlm.nih.gov/pmc/articles/PMC5010718/
[19] https://dune.une.edu/cgi/viewcontent.cgi?article=1095&context=pt_studcrpaper

say that yoga poses are quite useful when pain reduction and functionality are the required or desired effect!

So, to do this pose, follow the steps below:

- First, warm-up.

- Have a seat and take a pair of weight dumbbells. If you have a resistance band, then that this okay too. If you intend to use a band, consider sitting on it or sliding it under the chair. Ensure you keep it at an equal length on either side of your body.

- When seated, ensure you are comfortable. Your hips should be as far back as possible, with your back firmly placed on the chair's backrest.

- Tighten your core.

- Spread both elbows to the sides of your body.

- Align both elbows under your shoulders and stick your chest out.

- Place your palms forward and grip your dumbbells.

- Raise your arms. Extend them as much as possible but ensure that you feel no pain during the movement. Ensure that the arms are parallel and that the hands do not touch each other. Hold this position for 10 seconds or more.

- Slowly bring down your hands slowly to your original position. While bringing the hands down, keep your elbows spread, elbows untucked, and not in the middle of the body.

- Do a minimum of 10 repetitions.

Seated Yoga Exercise 8: Seated Front Shoulder Raises

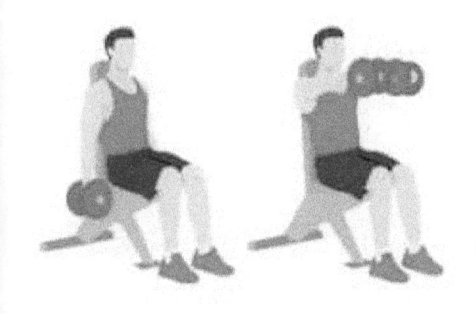

This pose will target your biceps, upper chest muscles, and the fronts and sides of the shoulders.

In the last pose, we saw what shoulder issues you are most likely to have and what steps you should take to strengthen the shoulders, remember? In addition to helping you avoid shoulder-related illnesses, this pose will help you avoid muscular dystrophy, bicep tendonitis, asthma, heart disease, chronic obstructive pulmonary disorder, respiratory tract infections, hypoxia, hypercapnia, sarcopenia, etc.

Several studies have proved that this pose will help your upper body. They are:

A study conducted in 2019 titled "Positive effects of yoga on physical and respiratory functions in healthy inactive idle-aged people[20]" says that eight weeks of yoga (in this case, the seated front shoulder raises) will boost respiratory functions and improve inspiratory muscle strength and global body flexibility.

Another study conducted in 2015 titled "Effects of a 12-week hatha yoga intervention on cardiorespiratory endurance, muscular strength and endurance, and flexibility in Hong Kong Chinese adults: A controlled clinical

---

[20] https://www.ncbi.nlm.nih.gov/pmc/articles/PMC6329219/

trial[21]" says that a 12-week yoga exercise (in this case, the seated front shoulder raises) will help boost cardiorespiratory endurance and muscular strength, flexibility, and endurance.

So, to do this pose, follow the steps below:

- First, warm up.

- Place a pair of dumbbells, medicine ball, or resistance band, then have a seat.

- Tighten your core.

- Stick your chest out.

- Pick up your dumbbells, then keep your arms resting on your body's sides. Ensure your arms hand with both palms facing towards the body.

- If you will be using a resistance band, slide it under your seat or sit on it.

---

[21] https://www.ncbi.nlm.nih.gov/pmc/articles/PMC4475706/

Ensure that the band is at equal length on both sides of the body. Keep both arms to the sides of your body and let them hang with your palms facing towards the body.

- If you will use a medicine ball, place it at the edge of your lap, then keep your hands on either side while you grip the ball.

- Have your palms facing the opposite direction and your arms straight.

- Move the arms up in front of the body.

- Slowly return to the original position.

- Do a minimum of 10 repetitions.

You can also do arm raises on the couch. To do so, follow the steps below:

For this yoga pose, you will need to have some weights. You can use bottles of wine.

- First, warm-up.

- Get a couch and sit with while the back is straight.

- Slowly lift the bottles of wine out to the side. Lift them until your arms are parallel to the floor as high as possible without getting hurt.

- Hold this position for 20 seconds.

- Lower back down again.

- Do 20 repetitions to complete the exercise.

Seated Yoga Exercise 9: Seated Chest Press

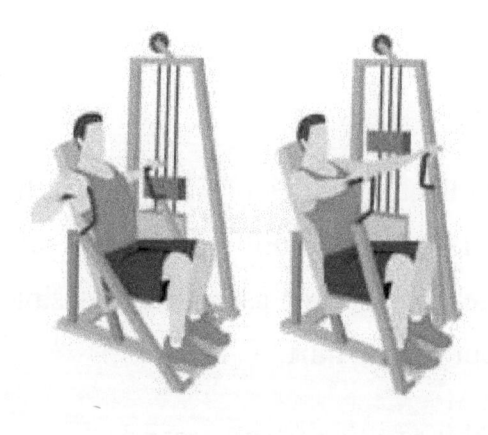

This seated yoga pose will target your triceps, shoulders, and chest muscles all at once, thus giving this yoga pose a unique name, "the compound movement."

In the previous exercises, we discussed which illnesses affect the shoulders and chest. Let us now look at what illnesses affect the triceps, shall we?

As a senior, you are at a higher risk of suffering from illnesses like tendinopathy or triceps tendonitis, subluxation, sarcopenia, amyotrophic lateral sclerosis, bicep tendon rupture, and others.

This means if you are suffering from acute pain due to an illness such as tendonitis, then doing this yoga pose will come in handy. Proof of this is in a study titled "Effectiveness and safety of yoga to treat chronic and acute pain: a rapid review systematic reviews[22]." This study shows that engaging in yoga will help take care of any back and cervical pains, which is quite helpful for senior adults.

---

[22] https://www.ncbi.nlm.nih.gov/pmc/articles/PMC8719171/

So, to do this pose, follow the steps below;

- First, warm up.

- Grab a resistance band.

- Place your resistance band behind your back (where the shoulder blades would be). Please ensure that the resistance band does not move on the back of the chair because this will increase the chances of injury or exercising the wrong muscles. To keep it secure, you can use a pin or clip. You can also get help from someone (the person can install a couple of shelving brackets to the back of your chair. This will help position the band).

- Place your hips as far as possible.

- Ensure your back is firm and that it is placed firmly on the backrest of your chair.

- Tighten your core and stick your chest outwards. While doing all these, ensure you feel no pain at all).

- Keep your alms down.

- Keep your elbows bent and ensure that they are parallel to your shoulders.

- Position both hands outside of the shoulder width.

- Push your resistance band forward until you have your arms fully extended in front of the body. As you do this, be keen not to touch your hands together).

- Gently and slowly return to the original position.

- Do a minimum of 10 repetitions.

Please note that if you find it hard to place or fix the resistance band as instructed above, you have another choice: You can wrap the band around any firm post, such as a beam or a post.

You can also do this exercise from a couch. To do this, follow the steps below:

- First, warm-up.

- Sit on a couch.

- Have your arms stay parallel to the floor.

- Clasp your hands at the chest.

- Squeeze your palms together. While doing this, tighten your chest muscles.

- Hold this position for 20 seconds.

- Do 20 repetitions to complete the exercise!

Seated Yoga Exercise 10: Isolated Tricep Extensions

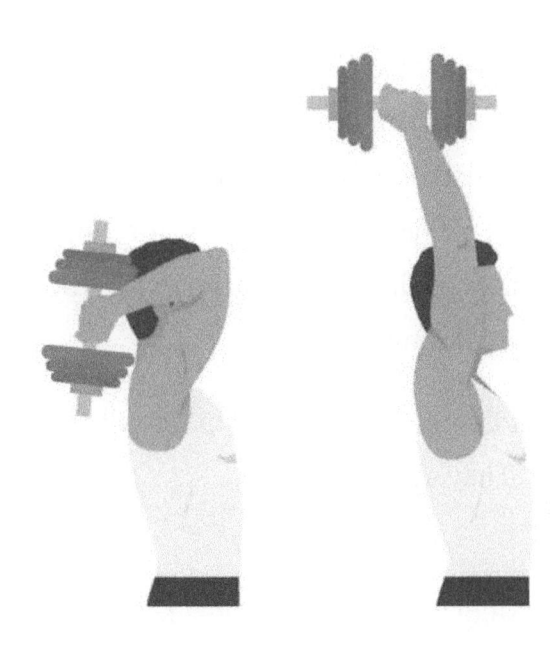

This pose will target your core, shoulders, and triceps (specifically, it will target the back of your upper arm). In previous sections, we discussed what affects the shoulders and triceps, so we will now discuss more about what affects the core.

As you may know, your core interconnects with different parts, such as the diaphragm, abdomen, glutes, hips, and pelvis. These parts are affected by illnesses and disorders such as sarcopenia, cardiac cachexia, Chilaiditi's syndrome, diaphragmatic paralysis or paresis, chronic obstructive pulmonary disease, chronic pelvic pain, pelvic ring fractures, decubitus, pneumonia, urinary tract infection, osteoporosis, among others.

Several studies prove that this pose will help your body. They are:

A 2022 study titled "The effects of yoga exercise of pelvic floor rehabilitation of postpartum women[23]" says that yoga (in this case, the isolated triceps extension) significantly improves your physical indicators and may also improve your mental health!

---

[23] https://www.ncbi.nlm.nih.gov/pmc/articles/PMC8808187/

For the diaphragm[24], it is essential to note that you need to begin working on it right away. Specifically, during the first two weeks of training, your diaphragm muscles will significantly improve their capacity to use oxygen after two weeks.

So, to do this pose, follow the steps below:

- First, warm-up.

- Grab some dumbbells.

- Ensure you are quite comfortable in your sitting position. Your hips should be as far back as possible, and your back firmly pressed to the chair's backrest.

- Tighten your core and stick your chest out.

- Raise your elbows in front of your body.

---

[24] https://bit.ly/3IrZyaR

- Lower one hand behind your head. That should create a "V" shape

- Use the other hand to brace the arm under your elbow; hold this position for 10 seconds or more. However, be keen not to feel any pain while doing this.

- Ensure the hand holding the dumbbell has its palm facing the head.

- Raise the arm holding the dumbbell over your head until it is fully extended

- Gently and slowly lower your forearm back to the original position.

- Switch to the other hand and repeat the steps above.

- Do 20 repetitions or more.

Seated Yoga Exercise 11: Bicep Curls

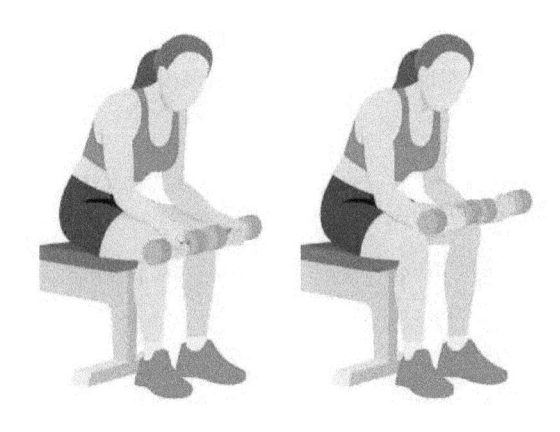

This yoga pose will target your forearms and biceps. We have discussed in previous yoga poses what illnesses affect these two parts and proof that yoga truly helps. The only remaining thing is to learn how to do this exercise. Let us do this next:

- First, warm-up.

- Grab a resistance band or a pair of dumbbells.

- For a resistance band, have it go under what you are sitting on or sit on it. Ensure that the length is equal on both sides.

- Sit such that the hips are kept or placed as far back as possible. In addition, ensure that your back is firm to the chair's backrest.

- Tighten your core and stick your chest out.

- Keep both arms to the side of your body and let them hang with both palms facing forward. Ensure you keep your elbows tucked to the sides of your body.

- Move both forearms. Ensure to do this in a curled-up motion. Start from the sides of your body, then move to the front of the shoulders. While doing this, you do not have to touch your hands to your shoulders for you to experience a full range of motion.

- Keep the tension and gently and slowly lower both your forearms back to the original position.

Seated Yoga Exercise 12: Knee-to-Chest Pose

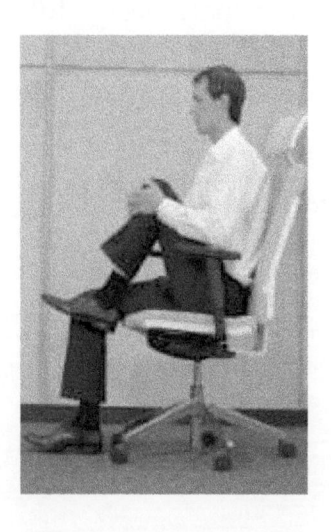

This pose will target your lower back muscles primarily. Specifically, this pose will target your buttocks, glutes, and hip flexor. We have discussed the effects that affect these different parts and proof that seated poses work. The only thing left now is to learn how to do it.

Let us do this next, shall we?

- First, warm-up.

- Sit comfortably at the edge of your chair. Do this without feeling like you are falling over.

- Straighten and tighten your back and core. In addition, stick your chest out too.

- Place your feet in front of you as much as possible and point your toes upwards. Ensure your hips are diagonal to your hips.

- Raise both your legs and bring them closer to your body.

- Bend your knees. While bending the knees, go as close to the chest as possible (do this with both knees).

- Follow the steps above but this time, do it in the opposite direction. Do this until you get to your starting point. This will be the end of one repetition.

- Do a minimum of 10 repetitions to complete the exercise!

Seated Yoga Exercise 13: Seated Ts

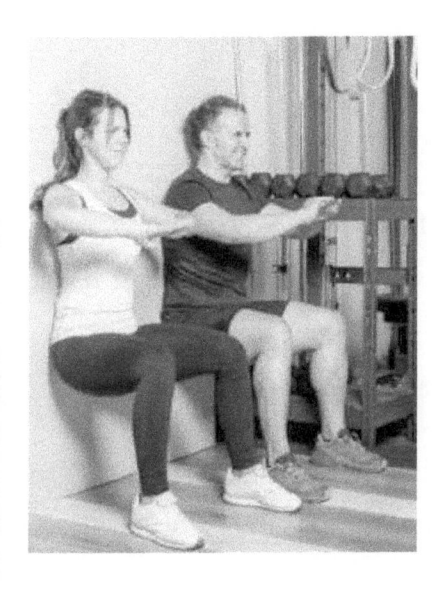

This yoga pose will target your upper back and shoulders. As discussed in previous yoga poses, various illnesses and disorders can affect these two parts and proof that yoga will help. So, without much further ado, let us learn what steps are involved in doing this pose, shall we?

- First, warm-up.

- Get a seat and sit with your feet wider than shoulder-width apart.

- Extend your hands.

- Keep your back straight.

- Bend forward.

- Stick your fingers outwards, then raise your hands. Go as high as shoulder level. Hold this position for at least 10 seconds, then bring them down.

- Do a minimum of 10 repetitions to complete the exercise!

Seated Yoga Exercise 14: Seated Leg Scissors

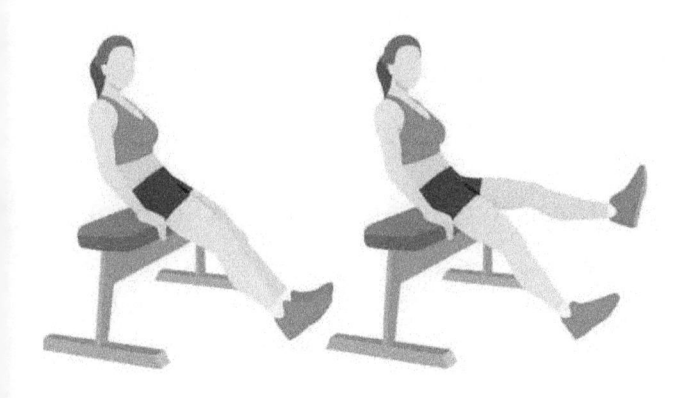

This couch yoga pose will target your abs.

We have already discussed what affects the core and proof to entice you to adopt yoga. Do you remember?

Well, with that in mind, let us learn how to do this couch yoga pose, shall we?

- First, warm-up.

- Get a couch/sofa and put your hands on your body in a way that seems like you are supporting your body.

- Have your legs straight out in front of you.

- Open and cross your legs. Do this at your feet. While doing this, alternate your legs while having them lifted off the floor.

- Also, while alternating your legs, tighten your abs and keep breathing as you continue your motion.

- And you are done!

Seated Yoga Exercise 15: Seated Crunches

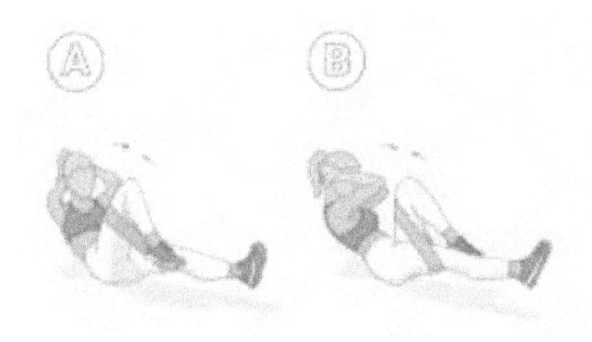

Seated crunches will also target your abdomen. As we have seen in previous exercises, some illnesses and disorders can affect this part. We have also seen (through studies) how yoga poses will help you.

Do you remember? With all this in mind, let us learn how to do this specific yoga pose.

- First, warm-up.
- Get a couch and sit on its edge.
- Grip the front of the couch's cushions with your hands.
- Extend your legs.
- Lean back. While doing this, ensure that your heels are around six inches off the floor.
- Gently and slowly bend your knees.
- Raise your legs towards your chest.
- Extend your legs.
- Finally, do a minimum of 20 repetitions.

Seated Yoga Exercise 16: Seated Chest Opener

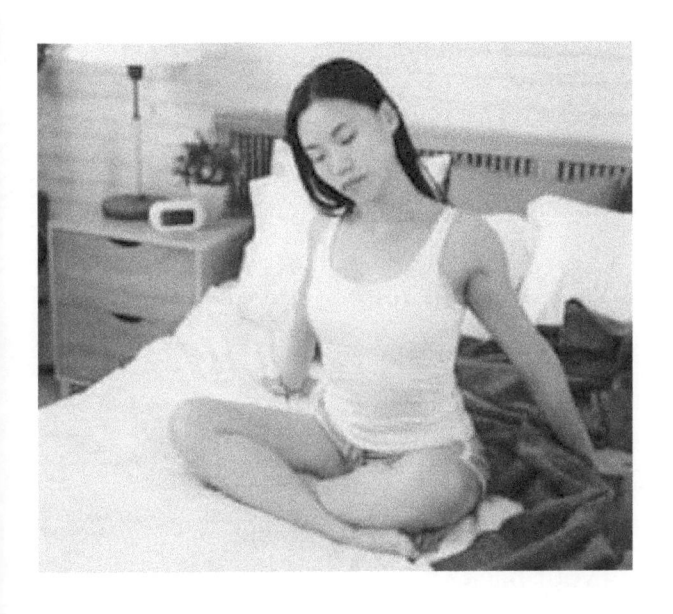

This yoga pose will target the front of your shoulders, torso, and chest muscles. In previous chapters, we saw what illnesses and disorders affect these parts. We also mentioned a few studies proving that yoga will help work these parts.

With this background information in mind, let us learn how to do this pose, shall we?

- First, warm-up.

- Get a seat and sit on its edge.

- Interlace your hands behind your back.

- Inhale and hold this position for a minimum of 10 seconds.

- While inhaling, lift your hands up.

- Have the hands positioned away from your back.

- Gently lift your chin away from the chest, then inhale.

- Hold this position for at least 10 seconds, then exhale while lowering your hands.

- Do 20 repetitions to complete the exercise!

Because we have covered a healthy selection of seated yoga poses that target the upper body, we can focus on the lower body:

Lower Body Seated Yoga Exercises

While exercising the upper body is important, do not forget to exercise your lower body because it will help you move easily from one place to the other and keep illnesses such as diabetes, heart illnesses, and arthritis at bay.

Since we have discussed different seated exercises that target your upper body, let us list and discuss different exercises that target the lower body.

Seated Yoga Exercise 17: Chair Warrior

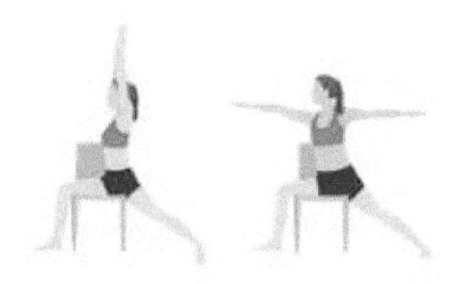

This pose, better known as a hip opener, will target your legs (front and rear thigh) and the upper arms too! This pose will also elevate pains and tension from illnesses associated with these two body parts:

- **Legs (front and rear thigh):** You will feel less pain and discomfort from leg illnesses and disorders such as restless legs syndrome, leg cramps, pinched nerve, stroke, Guillain barre syndrome, spinal tumors, Parkinson's, and amyotrophic lateral sclerosis. Proof of this is in a study titled "The effects of yoga on pain, mobility, and quality of life in patients with knee osteoarthritis: A systematic review" in 2016[25]. The study proves that yoga poses, in this case, chair warrior, may positively affect your life. Specifically, this stretch will help relieve pain and boost mobility.

- **Hips:** You will feel less pain and discomfort from hip illnesses and disorders such as wear and tear arthritis, developmental dysplasia, Perthes disease, irritable hip syndrome, soft tissue pain and referred pain, and slipped capital femoral epiphysis. Proof of this is in a study done in 2016 titled "A

---

[25] https://www.ncbi.nlm.nih.gov/pmc/articles/PMC5061981/

pilot randomized controlled trial of the effects of chair yoga on pain and physical function among community-dwelling older adults with lower extremity osteoarthritis[26]." This study proved that seated yoga, in this case, the chair warrior pose, will help reduce hip pain.

To do this pose, follow the steps below:

- First, warm-up.

- Next, sit on your seat.

- Face forward.

- Place your arms by your side.

- Spread your hands and lift them wide apart, as shown in the image above.

- Place one leg across the chair, then turn your torso forward. Kindly note that this

---

[26] https://agsjournals.onlinelibrary.wiley.com/doi/abs/10.1111/jgs.14717

is an optional step you should try to do until the point you feel slightly uncomfortable.

- Next, inhale and raise your arms towards the ceiling. At this juncture, hold your position for 5 seconds minimum.

- Next, exhale and lower your arms to the original position.

- Next, put your legs together, switch your feet, and repeat all the steps above.

- Do 10 repetitions

Seated Yoga Exercise 18: Eagles Arms

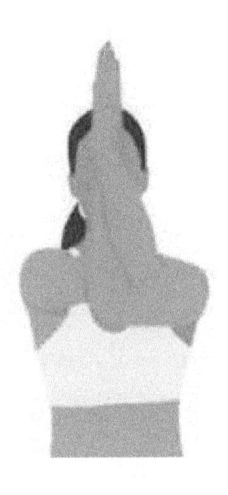

This pose targets your fingers, elbows, calf, thigh, and knees. Therefore, this pose will alleviate pains and tension from illnesses associated with these six body parts:

- **Fingers:** You will feel less pain and discomfort from finger illnesses and disorders such as rheumatoid arthritis, osteoarthritis, Parkinson's, and hand osteoarthritis. Proof of this is in a study titled "Expectations and effects of a single yoga session on pain perception[27]." This study urges us to consider yoga as a long-term practice if we need to see finger and other joint pain reduced drastically. Given this, you can benefit from adopting seated yoga as a long-term option if you want to enjoy its full benefits.

- **Elbow:** You will feel less pain and discomfort from elbow illnesses and disorders such as rheumatoid arthritis, lupus, and gout. Care24, a renowned world care home,[28] proved this in their report that says yoga poses directed specifically on the elbow will reduce pain levels and help lower elbow inflammation.

---

[27] https://bit.ly/3Ghl7rT
[28] https://care24.co.in/blog/3-yoga-exercises-for-tennis-elbow/

To do this pose, follow the steps below;

- First, warm-up.
- Next, get a seat and sit on it.
- Next, slide back and sit upright.
- Stretch your arms in front of you and cross the left arm over the right.
- Next, bring your elbows together. To do this, bend your elbows and
- Slightly interlace your fingers.
- Raise your elbows slightly. Do it until you feel your back arch.
- Hold that position for 10 breaths, each being 5 seconds.
- Finally, return to the original position and switch the arms.

Seated Yoga Exercise 19: Seated Forward Bend/ Paschimottanasana in Sanskrit

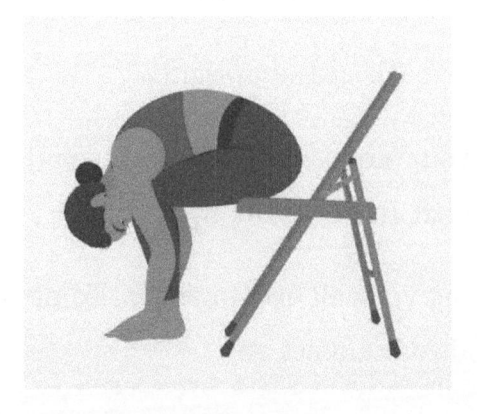

This pose targets your lower back muscles, hip flexors, glutes, calves, spine, and hamstrings. Therefore, this pose will elevate pain and tension from illnesses associated with these six body parts:

- **Glutes:** You will feel less pain and discomfort from glute illnesses and disorders such as glute tendinopathy, dead butt syndrome, and degenerative disc disease. Proof of this is in a study done in 2021 titled "Gluteal muscle activation during common yoga poses.[29]" The results of this study proved that yoga poses activate the glute muscles. Although yoga activates these muscles more in men than in women, it benefits both sexes.

- **Calves:** You will feel less pain and discomfort from calve illnesses and disorders such as anemia, Addison's disease, acute kidney failure, thyroid diseases, Parkinson's disease, osteoarthritis, nerve damage, muscle fatigue, involuntary nerve discharges, diarrhea, diabetes, cirrhosis, and chronic kidney disease. Proof of this is in a study done in 2021 titled "Effects of yoga exercises on diabetic Mellitus as

---

[29] https://www.ncbi.nlm.nih.gov/pmc/articles/PMC8168988/

validated by magnetic resonance imaging[30]." This study proved that yoga poses targeted at the foot produce a positive short-term effect and help with pain management. Thus, if you do it regularly, you might address the pain for good!

- **Hamstrings:** You will feel less pain and discomfort from hamstring problems such as tight hamstrings and strains. Proof of this is in a study titled "The effect of a hatha yoga practice on hamstring flexibility.[31]" This study says that a continuous 7-week yoga session – in this case, the seated forward bend– will improve hamstring flexibility and function, thus improving activities of daily living.

---

[30] https://www.ncbi.nlm.nih.gov/pmc/articles/PMC8023444/
[31] https://bit.ly/3X711Y3

To do this pose, follow the steps below;

- First, warm up.

- Sit on a chair, most preferably at the edge.

- Place your hands on the side of your body. Hold this position for 10 seconds.

- Lift your arms. Hold this position for 10 seconds.

- While lifting your arms, you can inhale and hold your breath for as long as possible. Start with 5 seconds but increase this time as you get accustomed to it.

- Exhale, then go down/bend. Start by bending and pausing at the waist, at the knees, then finally, as you touch your feet, as shown in the image above.

- As you go down, tighten your neck in one position to help avoid cranking up the spine.

- And you are done!

Seated Yoga Exercise 20: Marches

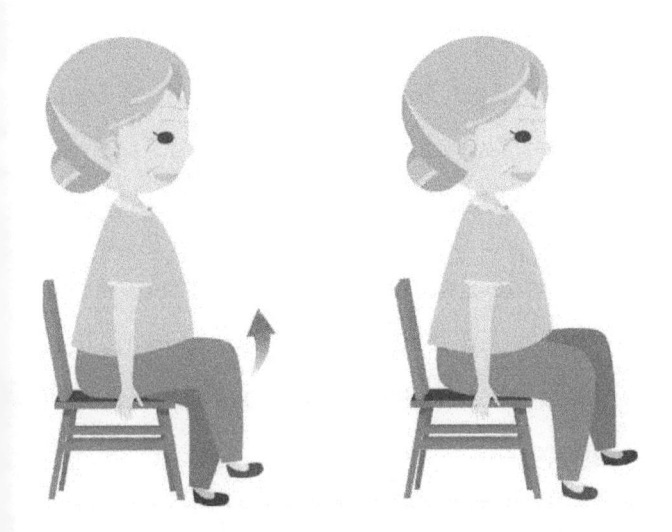

This pose targets your lower hip flexors and glutes (we have discussed what disorders and illnesses affect these parts and the proof that seated yoga poses in previous poses). So, to do this pose, follow the steps below:

- First, warm-up.

- Get a seat, couch, or bean bed, then sit upright. Ensure the feet are firmly flat on the floor. In addition, ensure that your back is away from the chair.

- Place your hands on the side of your body. You can also decide to go further and hold onto the chair.

- Lift one leg. When lifting the leg, make sure to lift it up as high as you can, then hold that position for 10 seconds or more.

- You can take a big breath when lifting up the leg to make this pose more intense. Exhale only when taking the leg down.

- Repeat the same steps with the opposite leg.

- For each leg, do 10 lifts.

To make this pose more challenging, follow the steps below:

- First, warm-up.

- Sit while the back is straight then proceed to ook forward,

- Curl your palms in such a way they form into fists.

- Have your hands placed on the chest level.

- Then proceed to raise your right hand.

- Lift one foot. While doing this, ensure that you flex your knee.

- Bring the knee up as high as possible.

- Bring your hand and leg back to the original position.

- Repeat the steps above using the other hand and leg. After you are done, this will be your one repetition.

- Do 2 sets of 20 repetitions to complete the exercise!

There is also another way of doing this. "How," you may wonder. Well, let us find out how through the steps below, shall we?

- First, warm-up.

- Get a seat and sit with your feet flat on the floor.

- Roll your shoulders back.

- Lift your hands and place them at the back of the head.

- Lift one foot and flex its knee.

- Crunch down. Do this in a way you aim at touching the right knee using your left elbow.

- Hold this position for 20 seconds, then return to your original position.

- Lift the other foot and follow the steps above.

- Do 2 sets of 20 repetitions to complete the pose!

There is still another way of doing this yoga pose. It is through another yoga pose known as the Couch Bike.

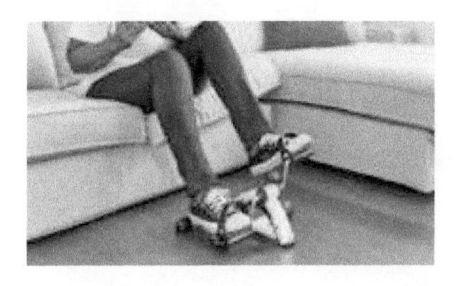

Kindly note that it is essential to try out the previous yoga pose first before advancing to this one because this one is slightly more intense.

With this in mind, follow the steps below to do this yoga pose:

- First, warm up.
- Get a couch, then sit while the back is straight and firm to the couch.

- Lift your legs. Have them positioned as if you are about to pedal a bicycle.

- Pin your legs as if you were pedaling a bicycle.

- Do 20 spins.

- You can also decide to hold your breath while pedaling. That will make it more intense.

Seated Yoga Exercise 21: Ankle Stretch

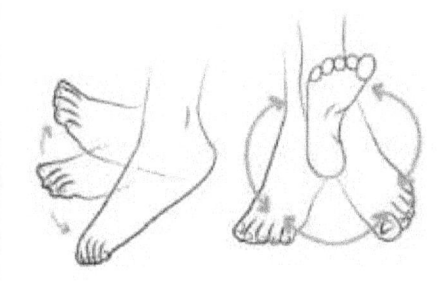

As the name suggests, this pose targets your ankles. Specifically, this pose will target all the surrounding muscles and tendons in and around the ankle area. So, if you have swollen ankles, gouty arthritis, edema, or cellulitis, among other ankle-related illnesses and disorders, this exercise/pose is for you!

You might be wondering, "How true is this? How true can this yoga pose help my ankles?"

Well, we can look to a study done in 2019 titled "Ankle motion in common yoga poses[32]" to answer that question.

This study proves that if you have had ankle surgery or have other ankle-related pain, yoga (in this case, the ankle stretch) will help reduce its pain, hasten the healing time and help you walk without pain again!

So, to do this pose, follow the steps below:

- First, warm-up.

- Get a seat, couch, or bean bed, then sit upright.

- Hold on to the base of your seat, couch, or bean bed, or simply put your hands on the side of the body.

---

[32] https://www.ncbi.nlm.nih.gov/pmc/articles/PMC7643884/

- Straighten one of your legs and raise it up from the floor.

- Point your toes towards you, then have them point away from you.

- Turn your foot area in circular motions. You can do 10 right circular motions, and 10 left circular motions. Once you get accustomed to it, you can increase the number of motions.

- Place your foot down on the floor, then repeat the steps above with the other foot.

- Stretch each foot 10 times or more.

Seated Yoga Exercise 22: Extender Leg Raises Pose

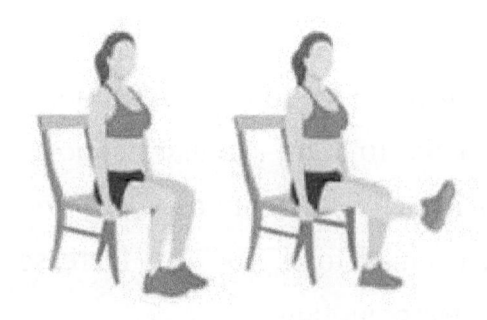

This seated yoga pose will target your anterior hip flexors, also known as the iliopsoas. Since we have already discussed the different illnesses and disorders that affect the hip flexors and proof that seated yoga will help, let us now discuss how to do this seated pose, shall we?

- First, warm-up.

- Get a seat and sit at its edge. Be careful not to fall over.

- Tighten your core and keep your back straight. In addition, stick your chest out.

- Place both arms at the sides of your chair.

- Grip your seat and try to be as stable as possible.

- Place your feet in front of your body

- Have your toes point to the ceiling. Kindly remember that both feet should be diagonal to your hips.

- Lift one leg and go as high as possible. Do the lifting without moving the center of your body. In addition, have the other leg stay in the original position.

- Return the leg to the original position. Go as slow as you can.

- Repeat the steps above with the other leg.

- Do 10 or more repetitions of this exercise.

This pose is the same as one yoga pose known as leg kicks. Let us look at how to do it:

Seated Yoga Exercise 23: Leg Kicks

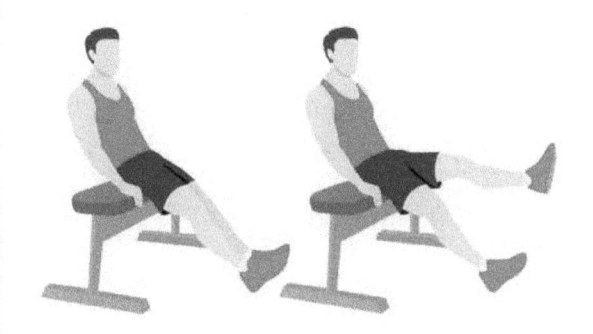

Here is how to do leg kicks:

- First, warm up.

- Get a seat and sit at its edge. Ensure not to feel like you are about to fall over.

- Straighten your back and tighten your core.

- Place your hands at the sides of the chair, then grip the seat; this will increase your stability.

- Place your feet in front of your body and have the toes point forward. Ensure both feet are diagonal to the hips.

- Lift one leg as high as possible. While doing the lifting, do so without moving the center of your body.

- Lower the lifted leg to the original position, then switch to the other leg. When switching the legs, lean your upper body backward for increased stability.

- Do 10 repetitions of the pose on each leg.

To make this and the previous yoga pose more challenging, do not touch the feet to the ground from the start to the end of the exercise. You can also decide to do the exercises in isolation– from one leg to the other. You only need to ensure you have the opposite leg firmly planted on the floor before doing any lifting.

You can also do this pose in another way that will yield similar results. To do this, follow the steps below:

- First, warm-up then proceed to lying on your side, as shown in the image above. Ensure your bottom leg, knee, and top leg are straight.

- Point your toes forward.

- Gently and slowly, raise your leg up as high as you possibly can. Raising the leg should start with the heel and then follow with the lower back.

- Hold this position for 20 seconds or more.

- Repeat this exercise on the other side, then do 20 or more repetitions.

There is still another way of doing leg raises. To do this, follow the steps below:

- First, warm-up.

- Go to a couch and lie on it face up with your legs extended.

- Have your palms facing downwards.

- Have your hands underneath your lower back.

- Raise your legs towards the ceiling. While you do this, keep your legs straight and press your thighs pressed together. In addition, keep your core and back tucked.

- Do not round your back off the couch.

- Raise your legs as high as you can.

- Finally, gently and slowly lower your legs down.

- Do 4 sets of 20 repetitions.

Seated Yoga Exercise 24: Knee Extensions

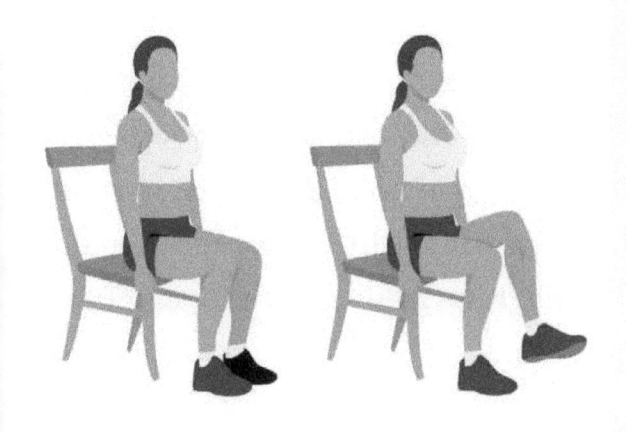

This yoga pose targets the front of your thigh: to be more specific, it will target your quadriceps muscle. You see, your quadricep muscle is under threat. You may be wondering, "Why?" It's because it is often at risk of illnesses and disorders like chronic obstructive pulmonary disease, knee osteoarthritis, sarcopenia, quadriparesis (also known as tetraparesis), and polymyalgia rheumatica, among others.

If you can recall, we dug deeper into the leg and thigh in previous yoga poses. Still, it is important to remind you through a study that yoga poses (in this case, the knee extension pose) will help you heal faster if you have any quadricep muscle-related issues, and if you do not, it will help reduce the chances of you getting them.

A study titled "Physical and perceptual benefits of yoga asana practice: results of a pilot study" done in 2005[33] involved 20 to 58 healthy adults to come up with encouraging results! The results of this study focused on dynamic muscular strength, upper body strength, diastolic blood pressure, among other things. Researchers noted that adopting yoga poses as

---

[33] https://www.sciencedirect.com/science/article/abs/pii/S1360859204000610

your ideal exercise (in this case, our focus is knee extensions) will help improve your trunk dynamic muscular strength, flexibility, and endurance. This proves that this pose will work!

Do you want to know how to do it? Well, follow the steps below:

- First, warm-up.

- Get a seat and sit comfortably.

- Place the hips as far back as possible. While doing this, keep your back firmly placed on the backrest.

- Tighten your core and stick your chest out.

- Have your hands (both of them) placed at the sides of your chair, then grip the seat. This will boost your stability.

- Have your feet sit at 90 degrees angle with the chair.

- Take one leg and extend it in front of you (take it upwards). Go as far as you can—if you can extend it fully, the better. While doing the extension, please keep the other leg right where it was when you started; this will add more stability.

- Hold this position as much as you can. Aim for 10 seconds or more.

- Gently and slowly as possible, return the extended leg to the original position.

- Switch to the other leg and follow the steps above.

- Do 10 or more repetitions for each leg.

Seated Yoga Exercise 25: Seated Hip Stretch

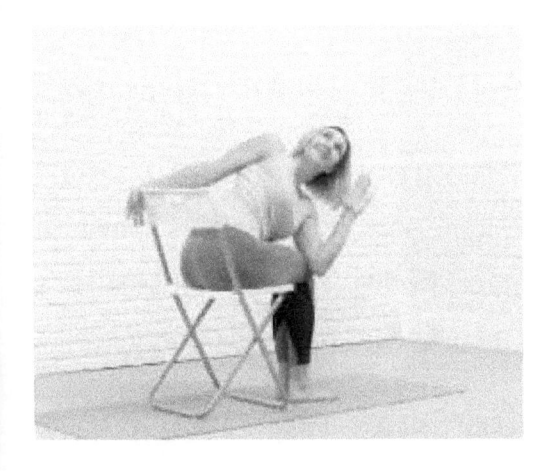

As this name suggests, this seated yoga pose will target your hips. As discussed in previous yoga poses, the hip is at risk of different illnesses. We also looked at several studies proving that the seated yoga poses we discussed can help your hips. Well, will this in mind, let us look at how to do this pose, shall we?

- First, warm-up.

- Get a seat and sit comfortably. Ensure your back is upright and that your spine is straight.

- Keep both feet firm and flat on the floor.

- Have one leg cross the other. This should create some sort of triangle, as shown in the images above. Push the crossed leg's ankle a few inches past the other leg.

- Bend your upper body forward. While bending, ensure your spine is straight, and your core is as straight as possible. Go far as you can, but stop when you feel some resistance in the glute or hip area.

- Hold this position for 20 seconds.

- Gently and slowly, bring the leg down, then shift to the other leg.

- Do 10 repetitions on each leg to complete your set! All you have to do now is increase the holding time after getting accustomed to it.

Seated Yoga Exercise 26: Seated Pillow Squeeze Pose

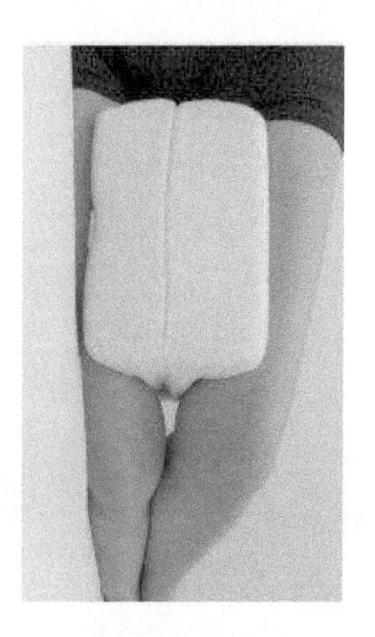

This Pilates exercise will target your pelvic floor muscles and the inner thighs. This means your pelvic muscles can suffer from illnesses and disorders like prolapse, dysfunction of sex, defecation, and micronutrition. For inner thighs, you might suffer from illnesses and disorders such as muscle strains, muscle dystrophy, hernia, and deep vein thrombosis, among others.

Different studies have proven that yoga can help deal with these two body parts and help alleviate pain. They include:

A study titled "A comprehensive review of yoga research in 2020" done in 2022[34] got information from over 4 studies that proved that yoga (in this case, the seated pillow squeeze pose) would help alleviate pain and address anxiety and postural balance!

Another 2022 study titled "The effects of yoga on pelvic floor rehabilitation of postpartum women[35]" reported that yoga (in this case, the seated pillow squeeze pose) helps strengthen the perineum muscles in females. In addition, it

---

[34] https://www.liebertpub.com/doi/10.1089/jicm.2021.0420
[35] https://bit.ly/3GGPmK2

will help prevent symptoms of lower urinary tract prolapse!

So, to do this pose, follow the steps below:

- First, warm-up.

- Seat down and place a pillow in between your knees. You can use a folded bed pillow or a small throw pillow.

- Have the legs parallel and the knees directly over the heels.

- Then proceed to squeeze the pillow using the strength of your thighs.

- Raise up on your toes and hold this position for 10 seconds or more.

- Do 20 or more repetitions.

Seated Yoga Exercise 27: Seated Clamshells

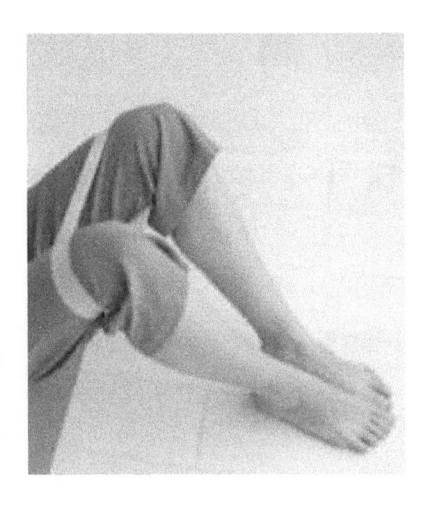

This yoga pose will target your gluteus medius, located on the outer edge of your buttocks. This means that some illnesses and disorders such as the gluteus medius syndrome, chronic lumbosacral and hip symptoms, gluteal tendinopathy, and many more that affect the gluteus medius will stop bothering you!

You still do not believe that yoga (in this case, the seated clamshells) has so much power? Well, studies back it up! For example, a study done in 2021 titled "Gluteal muscle activation during common yoga poses[36]" reports that yoga poses are perfect for activating the gluteus medius and the gluteus maximum. Kindly note that in this study, yoga activated the gluteus medius more in males and inexperienced persons than in females and experienced persons.

So, to do this pose, follow the steps below:

- First, warm-up.

- Seat on a normal seat or a bench. The trick is to sit on a firm object that is low enough to help you make a right-angle position.

---

[36] https://www.ncbi.nlm.nih.gov/pmc/articles/PMC8168988/

- Take a resistance band and tie it around both legs. Do this right above each kneecap, as seen in the image above.

- Sit in a way that keeps your back as straight as possible.

- Part your hands shoulder-width apart.

- Rotate your knees and push the band apart away from your body on both sides as far as possible.

- Finally, gently and slowly come back to the starting/original position. This is one repetition.

- Do a minimum of 10 repetitions to complete the exercise!

If you do not have a band, try following the steps below:

- First, warm-up.

- Get a chair and sit while the back is straight and arms resting on the side of the body.

- Bend your knees.

- Place your hands on the outside of the knees. You will notice that the hands will provide the needed resistance for your legs.

- Contract the outside muscles of your hips. To do this, move your knees away from each other. Always remember to use your hands to give you the resistance you need; all you have to do is push your knees inward.

- Hold this position for 10 seconds, then relax.

- Do a minimum of 10 repetitions.

You can also do this while lying down on the couch. To do this, follow the steps below:

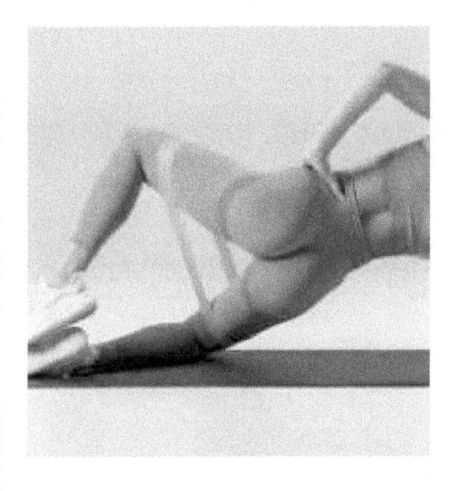

Although the image above shows our demonstrator not lying on a couch, you can do this yoga pose while lying on a couch.

Once you get a couch, follow the steps below:

- First, warm-up.

- Bend your legs and knees together.

- Raise your top leg as high as possible (this depends on the side you originally lay on).

- Lower your back down, then hold for 20 seconds.

- Repeat the steps above on the other side.

- Do a minimum of 20 repetitions to complete the exercise!

Seated Yoga Exercise 28: Seated Single-Leg Calf Raises

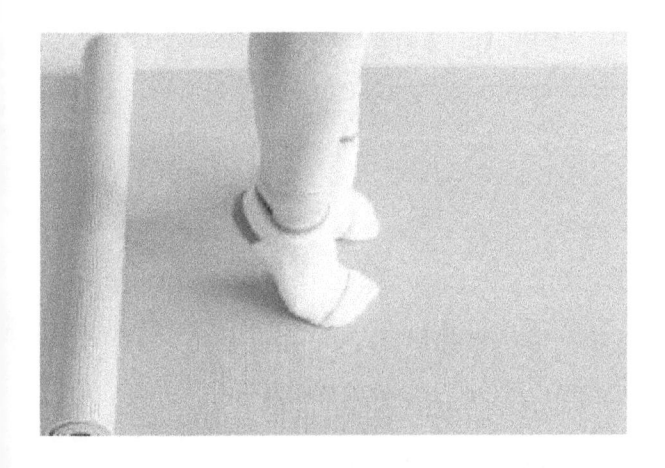

This yoga pose will target your tibialis anterior and the calf. It will also target a good part of the lower leg: the soleus and the gastrocnemius. Therefore, when you do this pose, you will avoid illnesses and disorders like the anterior compartment syndrome, spasticity, dystonia, tibialis anterior tendinopathy, bilateral calf chronic compartment syndrome, peripheral artery disease, sarcopenia, muscular dystrophy, edema caused mostly by chronic venous insufficiency, lumbar spinal stenosis syndrome, restless legs syndrome, and Guillain Barre syndrome among others.

To prove that this yoga pose can really help, let us look at some proven studies, shall we?

A 2011 study titled "The effects of yoga (Asana) on human lower limb muscles[37]" reports and affirms that yoga poses (in this case, the single-leg calf raise) will activate the tibialis anterior as compared to other exercises.

Another 2022 study titled "Harnessing the benefits of yoga for myositis, muscle dystrophies, and other musculoskeletal disorders[38]" reports and affirms that yoga poses will improve the overall quality of life and reduce morbidity if you are suffering from chronic illnesses.

---

[37] https://bit.ly/3Zg6qhh
[38] https://link.springer.com/article/10.1007/s10067-022-06280-2

So, to do this pose, follow the steps below:

- First, warm-up.

- Get yourself a tall chair and sit on it.

- Have your feet sit hip-distance apart, look straight ahead, then engage the core.

- Plant your feet on the floor.

- Lift one heel from the ground. Do this as high up as you can. While doing this, engage the calf.

- Hold this position for no less than 10 seconds, then lower the heel back to the floor.

- Do three sets minimum of 10 repetitions for each leg.

Once accustomed to one leg after the other, do three more sets of 10 repetitions where you lift both heels simultaneously. Once you reach the last set, hold the heels from the floor for a minimum of 20 seconds to close off the exercise!

Seated Yoga Exercise 29: Seated Beanbags Yoga Pose Routine

In the first chapter, we mentioned that you could also use beanbags. Do you remember? Well, let us see how. For this specific routine, we will use beanbags to boost visual motor integration, eye-hand coordination, and motor skills.

You see, visual motor integration is important. Are you curious about why? It is because this ability deteriorates as we age. Proof of this is in a study done by EC McNay and D.B Willingham titled "Deficit in learning of a motor skill requiring strategy, but no of perceptuomotor recalibration, with aging[39]" and another study done in 1994 titled "Rapid aimed limb movements: Age differences and practice effects in component submovements."

Eye coordination also declines as we age, which is why seniors often go through many adaptive eye-hand coordination challenges. A study titled "The effect of aging on adaptive eye-hand coordination" affirms it. This study's main conclusion is that perceptual-motor adaptability declines with advancing age[40]."

Last but not least, age also deeply affects motor skills. A study titled "Motor control and aging: Links to age-related brain structural, functional, and biochemical effects"[41] says that age brings along a decline in sensorimotor

---

[39] http://learnmem.cshlp.org/content/4/5/411.short
[40] https://academic.oup.com/psychsocgerontology/article/55/3/P151/607083
[41] https://bit.ly/3GJEcnV

control and functioning. These declines affect the daily life of every senior.

Here is what the above study had to say about this: *"These declines in fine motor control, gait, and balance affect the ability of older adults to perform activities of daily living and maintain their independence."*

With all these declines, you are probably eager to know how to do this specific exercise, right? Well, let us do this next, shall we?

Remember that this is a routine; it is also best to have a partner.

- First, warm up.

- Have you and your partner sit on chairs or couches; sit separately. Ideally, sit facing each other, about seven to 10 feet which is the same as 2 to 3 meters apart.

- Let one of you hold a beanbag.

- Have the one holding a beanbag throw it at the other one, and have the one without catching it with both hands.

- As the image above shows, have the one throwing the beanbag do so while twisting the body and using the opposite hand. For example, if the person throws it while twisting the body from the right, throw the pillow using the left hand.

- Also, have the one throwing the ball do so while holding their breath for a minimum of 5 seconds.

- Once the one receiving the beanbag does so properly without falling it or without feeling pain, continue doing the throwing and the catching 20 more times.

Seated Yoga Exercise 30: Seated Cow Face Pose

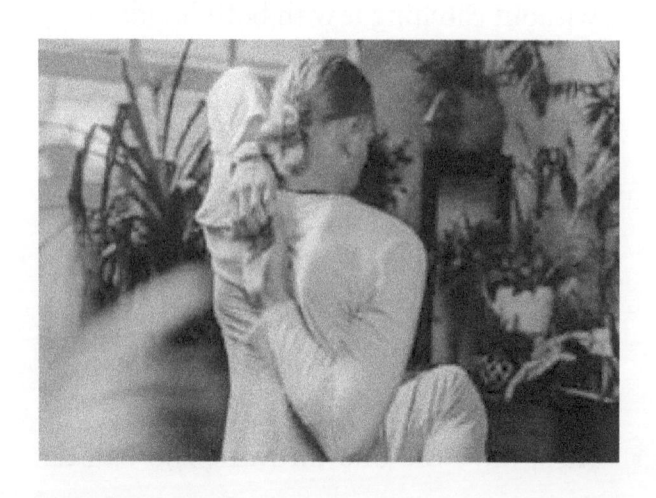

This powerful, seated yoga pose deep-stretches the ankles, hips, triceps, deltoids, and armpits. It also reduces chronic knee pain, clears the hip joint, decompresses the low spine, and strengthens your spine and the abdominals.

In previous exercises, we discussed the illnesses and conditions that affect these body parts and proof that the seated yoga pose helps, remember? So, without much further ado, let us learn how to do this exercise, shall we?

- First, warm-up.

- Sit on a chair or a couch.

- Get into a mountain pose with the cat/cow. We looked at how to do this in previous exercises.

- Hold that pose for 10 seconds or more, then go to the original position.

- Bring your legs and feet together.

- Lift one leg, preferably the right, and cross it over the left thigh.

- Extend your arms. They should be at your sides and parallel to the floor.

- Reach up with your left hand.

- Bring your bicep in line with your ear.

- Bend your elbow and reach your hand toward the back of your neck

- Rotate your right arm internally in a way your palms face behind you.

- Bend your right elbow.

- Bring the back of your hand towards your spine.

- Reach down with your left hand.

- Reach up with your right hand. The inching of both hands should be along the spine towards each other. Kindly note that your hands might meet at this juncture, but if they do not, this is still okay.

- Unwind and repeat the steps above on the opposite side.

- Do a minimum of 10 repetitions to complete the exercise!

Chapter 4: Seated Yoga Poses: A Few Things to Note

A common seated yoga question is, "How often should I do all these exercises?" Well, let us answer this.

How often should you do seated yoga poses?

The truth is that there are no set guidelines on how often you should practice chair yoga. What we can therefore rely on are the general guidelines the CDC gives.

The CDC says[42] seniors aged 65 and above should do two days of strengthening activities and three days of balance activities each week. From this, we can conclude that you should do

---

[42] https://www.cdc.gov/physicalactivity/basics/older_adults/index.htm

seated yoga two or three times every week as a beginner and then add to this as you progress.

How long should a seated yoga session be?

The best thing is to start small. A 30-minute seated yoga routine and then relaxing for 10 minutes will give you the desired benefits without pushing your body past the limits.

Conclusion

As this book has proven, seated yoga indeed works. Additionally, regardless of body type, abilities, or limitations, anyone can engage in chair yoga.

All you have to do is follow the steps this guide has outlined, exercise regularly, and watch your whole life change!

All the best!

PS: I'd like your feedback. If you are happy with this book, please leave a review on Amazon.

Please leave a review for this book on Amazon by visiting the page below:

https://amzn.to/2VMR5qr